Freebirth Manifesto

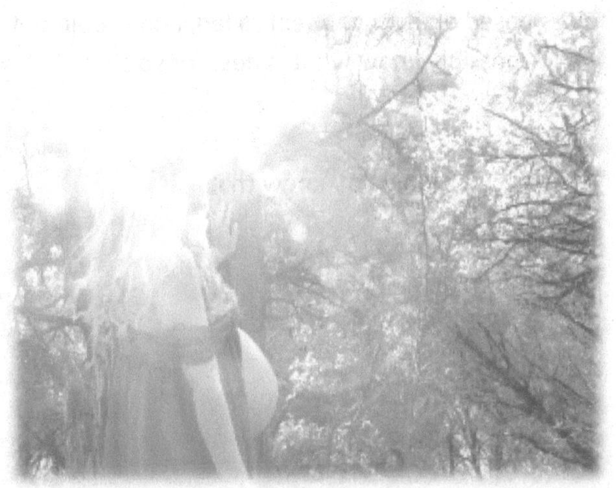

A True Story of Freebirthing at 44 Weeks

Faith ∞

Remember Who You Are.

This is a true story, but it is not a dictation for anyone else. This is my story. You need to make your own choices based on how you feel called, and I could not possibly know what is best for you.

Only You know that.

Any of the sharing herein is based on my personal journey. It is not instructive for somebody else to do as I have done.

Any freebirth is best done with at least one other adult present if that is the chosen path.

I personally feel that we need integrative care that's based on everybody's personal compass and reasonably rational choices paired with continual holistic self-care. The diet and habits of the average American creates a dependence on healthcare that is absolutely not natural nor needed. We can feel alive in every cell of our bodies through nutrition and basic self-care while abstaining from toxins. Easy peasey. If care is needed, it's available! We need more balance, more harmony. Right now, we need to interweave the ancient ways, including storytelling like this, and age-old wisdom, herbs, minerals, nutrients into a very intelligent and technologically savvy mechanized system that has gotten a little too much control a little too fast. All of it should be considered, all that is best should be used. We are that blessed.

∞

The timeline of this storytelling is perhaps as linear as it should be—not too much. Quantum Physics' view of the SpaceTime Continuum (not line) is more True than the average stories we get from the Western canon. So yes, I dive back into this storytelling several times over about a four-year span, and may again. Most of it is written during the pregnancy, but I am here throughout, editing in the future I knew would come all along. And sometimes I will add a thing or two and be pulled back into life and then jump right back in the deep end of this again. Because this is the biggest thing I have done in my life, and it's not well-approved of, and I am healing the people-pleaser version of myself back into the wild womban I am. For my Warrior Priestess daughters, I must try to live up to their standard and tell the story I promised to live and tell—not just live it, but tell it, too.

Sanctity of Birth

When we slow down during the natural process of labor, which begins with emotional labor, instead of keeping busy, and trying to rush through, we can come to a place of true appreciation for the sensations in fully knowing they are bringing the baby out into this world for us. In that level of expansive awareness, consciousness and presence, sensations never culminate into pain—instead they flow as their intent from God had designed them. And they actually expand naturally and become ecstasy. Birth becomes pleasurable in its entirety, even as the ebbs and flows of energy commence like a dance dancing through us and baby.

Fully experiencing and processing emotional labor leads to a transformational, fulfilling and successful birth process. Labor becomes a theme park ride. It becomes a wave we surf, flipping and loopdeelooing.

Other words for "labor": waves, birth process, a celebration. It's not work.

It's a gift that is given, a present that unfolds organically. Give it time, and time itself slows down through the process.

Birth is a rebirth.

As I write this, today is my birthday. I'm 36. Poetically, She—6 months now—sits beside me, awake at 4am on this rare occasion as if she knew I was talking about her and wanted to be in on it. We are immensely connected, because we have stayed connected, pregnancy through birth. No one has intervened. No one has touched the cord that connects me to her. Even when I physically cut her cord, I did so in love that saved the spiritual connection on such a level to preserve the gift of our natural mother/daughter bond.

It is sacred, and it lights up the world.

This is the power of connection between women and children.

This is my first time experiencing this kind of love. With my first daughter, that sanctity was taken from me. I love her equally, but the naturalness of it was intercepted and our entire relationship was affected, needing rebuilding, including her sleep and "colic."

My second now, this freebirth, has given me at least 8 hours of sleep almost every day of our lives together. She is so joyful. The sacred experience of respecting the birth portal and everything that comes with it has prevented postpartum depression this time unlike the last. Instead, I am reborn, too, with a new trust in my body and the miracle that is us. I am sovereign.

From day one, she is the smiliest baby I have ever seen. Every cell in us says "Yes" to this freebirth and always has since I first learned about it. I was enchanted. I just knew.

And that is not to say this path is right for everyone. But this is to say that it is right for everyone to follow their heart, trust their gut, and that includes absolutely everyone. It is key to get quiet, go within, and feel into each next step all along the way.

Please, let the one takeaway here be that you always, always trust your instinct. I am with you, whatever it is.

Feeling the baby move, reminds me of miracles. So much so that the whole world opens for me, and I believe in humanity again and again.

The Love that fills me in connection with my two children is far more than I can say. It flows so easily; they are loving me back so completely.

My partner and I have grown so much together and listened to one another in ways that helped us heal and thrive. Just like with my older daughter, we felt clearly when the time for our next child had come. And in about 3-4 months, we will see a sweet little face who surely will look like my older daughter and her Daddy and maybe not so much like me, which I predict and see as wonderful.

And much of this birth will be private in the sacred space. Just as I have waited so long to share the news of this pregnancy, not because of fear but because of Love. This is a rebirth for me, as this precious life blooms within me and I am blessed with the wisdom to really be here now, to know how important every moment of this journey is for me and our whole family.

Thank you for Loving us, supporting us, and honoring us at this special time.

12.14 (I posted this to a group)

Wild and free, feeling really open at 35 weeks. Who else has big life transformations during pregnancy?!?!? That human growth hormone is growing me, too, it seems!! Lowest lows and highest highs that are breaking through old family karma like never before. My dad passed just a month and a half ago and then things got really real. I processed it better because I dove in and have been doing the work for every generation. The timing was actually perfect. Right then I got two new mentors and my partner transitioned to the best job we could have ever wished for. It's weird I've been super active, even doordashing with my two-year-old, and I feel so empowered. Like this time the pregnancy is not just something to get through but something to lift me up. My body feels good and look at me, lol, nobody guesses I feel really good. Thank you for your wildness and wisdom to pave the way for women like me to know we can. Love you all so much. And I truly feel that what we are doing here is changing the world.

Yesterday we were hiking at a new place and the wind started blowing fiercely and my heart lit up and I just felt this portal we are in right now. I threw off my shoes and coat and asked my partner to take lots of pictures, because it was just a perfect moment. Here we are. A new birth for children, rebirth for us, and revival for the whole world. Wherever we are in our process, being here in this group is Divinely telling of leaps and bounds in the right direction. Grateful for you here now.

So inspired

12.24

I am safe

Baby is safe

I meet baby today

"my body was designed to birth," "yes I can open myself to the universe," "yes, I can open myself for baby to come through me"... the most recurrent was "I can open myself"

1.9.21

The tendency here, toward the 40 week mark of pregnancy, toward the end that leads directly into a new beginning, is to anticipate and reach for the next stage—the "result"—the post-natal, the baby.

However, that is not my intention as my pen touches this paper this 39th week when my baby is assuredly ready to make her debut and I am the one still blooming like a flower to open fully to the sacred portal I am now.

My intention is to be present. To be here and now.

I had asked my baby if she was ready two nights ago. She said, "yes."

But then I wondered, am I ready? She said she is waiting for me. I said, "how can I be ready?" she said, "how does a flower bloom?" It just happens in divinely right timing. In Trust. In the safety of Nature's all-encompassing embrace, the most delicate of treasures blossoms one petal at a time, or sometimes all at once in Symphony with her environment.

In synchronicity.

In harmony. In agreement with all that is.

And the rushing is not what's needed here now. It is the presence.

For while I know the privilege I am afforded and being educated in free birth, to release the chains of consumerism that bind the sad and sallow modern-day mother, I too know that this precious moment just before the flower fully opens is a delicate and unexplored one to be sure.

A full-size baby kicks within my womb. And that is what people see of me now. They look to the result. To it being "over yet?" "any day now?" "soon I hope."

And I don't want to be brainwashed by that rush. As adrenaline courses through me with each early contraction I Surrender into the arms of the biological birth keeper—this miraculous body, capable of such amazing things.

The placenta carries 1000 times the hormones of a regular woman. This baby is now being enlivened by Spirit right Within Me. The miracle occurs.

And it is a moment in time that lasts for eternity and only grows brighter in the sacred Silence of this presence.

This moment that so many rush is what gives life to the universe, literally and figuratively. It is a moment we need to story.

The waves of emotions rise up to precede the physical sensation of the waves that open the body. They are a spiritual practice.

A wave of fear.

Come into Trust.

Release.

Healing swells over.

A pull of longing for this baby to come. And a remembering- -she is already here. Partner in symbiosis. Witness and assistant and even director in oscillation from her wisdom to mine in the conversation of our ancient forms together.

A Stillness amongst chaos. A feeling of being in the eye of the storm and rising to new heights for all of existence. Quietly saving the world, without expectation for acknowledgement and yet deepest commitment to the voice of the ancient divine feminine that has been silenced for long enough. No more. No more silence. No more waiting for approval.

This.

This fiery icy sureness that all is well Within Me is what is needed now.

And to let will subside to Divine will. So that the rising Waters Within Me swell to Encompass the hearts of those who had been captive before, by a barbarous, taking commercialism.

release.

release.

Release.

The Secret of women—all women—is that we have always been this powerful. It is the gentlest and most powerful force on Earth to be a woman. And awakened men know this, honor, and do everything to support it. They walk with us only as far as they can go and then they Trust. And God is with us as the baby takes shape and the baby emerges through us. It's all an evolution. And I take back my role in it. I take it back for all of us women. I give it back to all of us women now. In this quiet moment so rare to witness. Before the storm and within it. The waters rise and part.

[Looking back at this in June of 2024, seemingly random spaces appeared. But I notice this pattern, and a message in the areas with an extra space if you read the underlines words:

The Secret of women--all women--is that we have always been this powerful. It is the gentlest and most powerful force on Earth to be a woman. And awakened men know this, honor, and do everything to support it. They walk with us only as far as they can go and then they Trust. And God is with us as the baby takes shape and the baby emerges through us. It's all an evolution. And I take back my role in it. I take it back for all of us women. I give it back to all of us women now. In this quiet moment so rare to witness. Before the storm and within it. The waters rise and part.

As written here: "Always been powerful force, know this, with us God is in it. Us women."]

For God is with us.

And the journey is the reward.

And this baby is changing the world.

Already. Like you.

And like me.

And most of all, together.

The True Quiet.

The Solace inside the heartbeat of my soul. When my two-year-old is napping, and all is finally still, that I might rest my muscles and bones that shape clay into being. Definitely and certainly peer out of the hidden window into a world but half the world may glance but once or twice—or more, if granted. The regenerative gift of natural birth.

A sip of chamomile lavender tea, warm and soothing calming to the nerves that forget to surrender just before. And welcoming and Trust. Remembering. Remembering my place as a woman. My true place. My throne. My hilltop on which to preach. My Mountain to Summit and breathe deeply the air of My Success. And to most of all remember the breaths given now, in this moment—the life-giving ones.

Rivers of light flow through me now. Many people see it in my eyes—a silent part of them acknowledges and delights in this sacred presence through me and among them now. They nearly squirm at the meeting of my warm aura with theirs. Everyone knows—even the ones who think too much.

Birth is Joyful ♥

Affirmations ♥

I love giving birth!

My body is capable of amazing things.

My baby is wise.

My body is wise.

This baby and this body are wise.

My baby will choose the perfect time for her birth.

There is only one sensation, after that one I'm given time to rest.

I trust!

Soon I'll be holding my baby, feeling only love and ecstasy. Birth is joyful.

My body opens like a flower.

My cervix is opening like a flower.

The universe has room for the love I have for my baby. My baby is healthy whole and safe.

I am healthy whole and safe

I cut all cords and dissolve all contracts with any being or entity whatsoever not the best, so that the baby's birth can happen in the most beautiful free birth way. Just to be loved. Permanently and completely. And

replace and simultaneously dissolve any remaining not
the love with love of God now and forever.

Herbs for Birth

(HERBS MANY USE FOR FREEBIRTH, AND I WISH I WOULD HAVE HAD AT MY FIRST BIRTH. I used them effectively at my freebirth.):

HERBAL TINCTURE REFERENCE AND DOSAGE (from unassisted / freebirth fb page)

(tinctures can be found at Inhishands.com online store)

Angelica: used for heavy bleeding before the placenta is delivered. Can also be used for slow to deliver placenta. Tincture is best. 30-40 drops or a half vial every few minutes if post birth and heavily bleeding. should be left under the tongue for 1 seconds and only have a small amount of fluids to rinse mouth. do NOT dilute. Can also be used for retained placenta or bag even if its days after the birth. Take hourly in this case.

Wombstringe: has shepherd's purse in it and stronger than the single herb. Used for bleeding after the placenta is birthed. tincture best. 40 drops or a half vial under tongue for 10 seconds before swallowing. do not dilute. Can be taken every few minutes until bleeding stops. Can also be used for prevention of bleeding after birth of placenta as well.

Mantra (read again when fears arose on 2/2)

Releasing the thoughts that arise. Many of them are just things others have said in fear, and they are not true. I release and find peace and calmness, power and true right knowing as I'm grounded back into living flowing undulating waves of trust and divinely-guided organic and creative experience.

At a prenatal Circle, we women shared a single red thread, a strand woven around are with wrist three times, one for Grandma, one for mother, and one for ourselves, and ancestral connection, Divine Connection, and communal light—together we vowed to wear the Strand until my baby came to Earth side—her name is the same as my Grandmother's, so it truly is the completion of the circle, coming full circle, a circuit closing as a new life opens.

I wear those strands now, and I'm supported by my sisters and mothers who wear them too. I feel the fibers on my soft skin. The fit was exact in my arm has stayed the same size because of the commitment to help I've made in this birthing. And I see, that my bracelet came out with 4 strands. Perhaps the fourth layer is for my daughters to, who mother me as I am reborn with them, with my older daughter wants, and now again my flower blooming to great new depths with the birth of the second mother, this child who connects my family line—grandmother, two daughters daughter. Who closes the circuit and opens the flow of creative force that flows through us now, as one. One family of women, pulsating with Divine Mothers' Light as One.

A flock of birds flew overhead today. Only one of the birds in the middle had white Wings. They move like water altogether. Like how music would look if it could be seen.

Was that White Winged Bird [Her]? So supported and so surrounded by The Divine Network.

Together We rise.

The many birds that moved like water remind me of supporting ancestors and so, too, all the women here on Earth, and beings who helped. We, the great Symphony, can only play our part, when we forget all else, and remember the truth of who we once were and are now, once again. Living memory.

Everything that's needed in life can be learned in the birth Journey. Bejeweling us with Timeless wisdom.

So much of who we are here to become and be meets Us in the birth portal for both mother and child alike.

1.10.21 1:27am

I didn't want to be like them. Because I needed to be me. And for that I would have to forget they existed as they. so all could become we.

Breathing

Deeply

Remember

Breathe it out.

Breathe it all out.

And enjoy the peace

of open spaces.

I write in the dark now. it must be close. ♥

Thank You ♥←

(2/2/21 just wrote this affirmation then opened to this!!!!!)

Lots of energy courses through me. I feel lit with truth. Do not even try to say anything but authentic truth around me. I am so open. I feel it all and just know. That's why our birth space and those we invite within are so important. They change our atmosphere. I yes. Peace and knowing. And rest in The Surety.

A guide or Angel showed me in a dream. I need to breathe deeply during the birth, and I felt the life-giving nourishment of a deep breath. It gives life. Fluid love. Deep breath is like a full drink in water, to the thirsty—soothing, releasing, and vitalizing.

Like an empty space becomes complete by a force of life that changes black and white to full color, that alivens. Breathing in life, breathing out sensation, and thereby going deeper there in 2 we're healing occurs. For Generations.

The whole universe conspires to grant me this beautiful freebirth.

♥ opened in magical time—caterpillar to butterfly)

I am liberated from expectation, from any word, and person any pressure and so the pressures within are released in this luxurious spaciousness of sacred creativity.

1.10.21 (read again 1.30)

Birth is joyful. Birth is a gift. Birth is pleasurable. It is a portal. For transformation. It is natural drugs. The greatest trip. A journey into the ethers of ecstasy. It is why I welcome my baby and myself—reborn.

1.11.21

Rebirthing the Birth Process Together

This Birth has been bringing up patterns of addiction in
me. It is a-diction (without words)—failing to put words
or knowing to the perceived discomfort in me and
alternatively seeking outside distraction as a course of
escape from the present moment—as it is. I recognized
it clearly in a deep prayer with my partner that
thereafter much relief was experienced in my heart. It
was a feeling of "pills." I felt it as a child when I laid in
bed at night at a time when one or both of my parents
had consumed excessive pain relievers.

As a gifted and highly sensitive, empathic person, I have
always been gifted with experience thing a wider array
of stimulations than just the ones within my own form
and yet most likely when I do it is echoing some part of
me, too, that relates and resonates with the experience
from something in my past that is meant to bring me
into Higher Learning and deeper truths. A part of my
curriculum for this lifetime, assuredly.

When we are pregnant, we women all become more
like that, soap for me my experience is exponentially
heightened and that's why I can bring words to it. It is
so visceral, so clear and potent, so evident and obvious.
Certain people must be completely removed from my
field, by my choosing or my surrender and the
arrangement of the universe by a higher Good in order

to allow my full fruition at this time. I see that now. I know them when I feel them.

My father passed out of Earthly form almost 3 months ago, and upon this reflection makes me wonder if he left partially to provide me with the space for this new blossoming, in a final Act of love in this lifetime to make up for a life of misdirection and his own escapism from the experiences he did not choose to bring himself and presents with and thereby dissolves. That brings me love, comfort and relief—and Trust in the universe that conspired so diligently on my behalf.

The addiction he left unintentionally as a legacy is dissolving with me, and future and present lines are helping me to do the work necessary to release those patterns and allow them to be reworked for the creative forces of love.

This discussion has very much to do with the mainstream discourse and perception of birth as something to "get through" and "finish" and therefore escape.

In mainstream birth, Women are drugged, their children dragged from their wombs by secondary agents, when all along the very woman has the capability to births on her own—and for the presence of that experience in and of herself to transform her into who she really is,. Beginning in the way of that and the stalling and halting of that transformation is like tearing a chrysalis away from the caterpillar before the wings are formed. It is wrong and fills me with the Primal Rage And recommitment to showing through trust in my body and this baby that naturally, organically, the process of birth unfolds like the Petals of a flower. Every necessary knowing is being granted at the right time. And speculation is wholly unnecessary in 99% of birth experience this. The dependence on the will, want an intrusion of other non-Central family members is but another form of out picturing—of addiction—a dissolution of divine connection and prioritizing the mines conjectures over the actual, lived experience of the central presence and so the presence of the divine within the mother. We Trust the baby to be formed by God—fingers and toes, seeing eyes, smelling nose—and then when it comes to the simple Act of the mother releasing the baby into the world, we go to man as Authority? And I do mean man, as it is the toxic masculine presence that takes authority over such a sacred and meant to be secret Act. Not to be confused with the awakened masculine which is not only equally valid and beautiful as the feminine but extraordinarily helpful when left to his own devices.

What's more is that it all happens in surrender but something more than the release of a form from within a creative form is happening. A spirit is imbuing into a form in the most complete Integrity it has had and becoming a new lifetime what's the birth of this child. That is something the Incorporated birthing machine of man neither heeds nor in so much as acknowledges. And at what cost? The only way to know is to hear with open ears, heart, and mind the account of the unhindered woman, the woman agent who has holy birth to her children in the presence of God that no other authority raised higher. To replace the addiction of a birth machine with her addiction of truly accounting the empowering nature of nature itself, when trusted and cultivated. The children born of these women are special, too, as they do not need to spend their lives attending to and releasing the ancestral traumas of the generations before, as their mothers have already done that work.

What more will they accomplish then, to Usher this new light of inherent knowing into a world still hidden for its gems? We shall see, and listen and hear new diction— new (and ancient) Truths coming to Light, when the Presence is welcomed.

We go into perceived pain and find relief awaiting us within all along.

We make times for our mothers to express, authentically, their experience.

A woman who writes in the Holistic Stages of Birth (a next step of reading for those who listen now) said that when a woman says, "I can't take this anymore" during birth—the key word is "this." That does not mean the only solution is chemical—as many doctors assume. "This" can be easily altered by movement, massage, smelling soothing oils, bathing in warm waters and so on...And now that I realize this, those are not medical but they are chemical, for the body naturally emits endorphins and pleasurable relaxing hormones especially through the birth portal and also before (as relaxin is naturally released to open the hips, human growth hormone floods the system to help create the baby, and so on)... The key here, is that our bodies are naturally equipped, and when we TRUST in us that is when both the best results and the most enjoyable process unfold through birth.

Well 30% of hospital births results in a c-section, 2% of home births do. Most women who have a truly uninterrupted home birth have minimal to non-existent tearing—the body when left to their own devices knows how to open gently for baby, and actually does it on its own through FER (fetal ejection reflex). Everything that the body does to construct the baby, it is capable of doing to birth the baby, as the birth is a continuation of the prenatal-natal postnatal cycle...

If some mind trapping does interrupt, then the gentler approach solving it would be holistic or herbal remedies—not barbaric physical manipulations or toxic medicines. Have tried and ignorant of this medical system always tied into profit.

As a note, the father modern birth medicine was first ever given dead bodies with which two experiment his findings. That is the foundation of medical birth practice—death. How unreliable and backward! Completely illogical proceed from a holistic standpoint.

This is New Life—precious experience that gives life to all involved when allowed to bloom. Taken image of a flower then. Can it be made to bloom simply by pulling each one of its pedals outward at the time when some farmer says the bloom is due? A baby's due date is simply an average of when half women tend to birth before and half after, and yet that is not in a vacuum with any constant variable available. That is with a certain percentage of the medically induced and forced births included, third which were cut from the body this is simply ignorant, outdated, and wildly inappropriate system, riddled with bullying and lie.

Women need to be educated and giving real choice— which I was not and am now.

And let us compare the two birth experience, whenever God chooses for this next little light worker to come into the Earth's ever transforming atmosphere. And let us see how we transform it together this time. And let it show how truly beautiful joyful and surrendered birth can be.

"Trusting guidance to come"

Birthing instructions manifest in the process! We do not know everything beforehand, but we can be sure the guidance will come whenever needed and will help us through the whole journey of breath.

Today I went to a park and a lovely lady with a "designer dog" let my older daughter chase and play fetch with this dog for ages; it was perfect—got her energy flowing and mine, too. And so joyful. As we left, I saw her get into the car parked behind mine and free us up for going back in perfect timing.

I smiled and felt joyous peace, back to the car up a bit, and while I had planned to move forward and go around the whole island in front of me, I realize that moment the instruction. But I had the space and capability to move over a complete donut U-turn and shorten the commute in the lot significantly. I just knew when the option became available—peacefully and divinely guided. It's a small thing that translates in big ways.

That's how it happens in an undisturbed birth. We know to move our bodies just so and make just such adjustments to improve the whole journey. And we accept ourselves in the driver's seat to take the initiative when guided so the inner voice is not muddled and instead remains clean, clear and easy to receive.

All along in birth, we are getting the cues and that continues with the birth process and can be just as enjoyable as the pregnancy itself ♥

(1.11 Trusting, 11pm)

Tomorrow is the baby's first due date.

I just found the spirit babies book again and in rereading the birth shaman part :)

[Inserted from 2.2.21

♥Open♥

Sparkling, glittering, twinkling light,

You make time stand still

No matter day, no matter night

You will come when we feel right.

Cosmic traveler, more than seen,

Lifetimes together, our hearts reborn,

A perfect moment comes to mean

We are found in light, two heart Sparks beam.]

"Dark Night of the Soul"

I'm feeling a potent rage and fear coming—primal. So much indignation that I have to do this much work to try to avoid torment and torture—but every person closest to me has a wound they're unconsciously trying to recreate in me—to show that they did nothing wrong by their choices by making me pay for my attempt at freedom. And are these two versions of myself of which I speak as well? Is there an internal me—the unconscious programming that pushes forward at all costs just to be "right" for all I have done?

I release her now, I release her from the bonds of perfection, past, present and future. I release her from whatever contracts may have bound her to recreate the un alive. I free her to the Liberty of authentic and natural birth.

This emotional pain is so potent. I must go within it. I must accept myself for it and forgive myself and all others for its appearance now. That is the only freedom. This is emotional labor. I'm sure of it. But I've never heard of it before. Breathe deeply—in healing—out fully—releasing all this extra. And I start to feel the natural drugs for my body rise to calm and euphorize my brain. My heart rate calms. I feel the tiredness that was behind the emotion now. The needed rest without stimulation. My teeth are gritted. Or at least my jaw and neck and heart.

"I honor the birth showman within me, I will act according to her wisdom" Spirit Babies

I saw her last night with feathers in her hair.

A specter lurks in hidden places in my mind and body. When I open, I see it. His name is "Hospital". It is eight letters. And the meaning is not. I let go of any meaning, and any true knowing of those eight letters. I release it for myself. My being. My past. My future. My family's past and future. My present. Released.

Birth is joyful. Birth is calm. Birth Is wild. I am being instructed now.

I can trust the process of birth ♥

I honor the birth shaman within me. I will act according to her wisdom.

Do not idolize the broken ones, the victims. That's what the transgressors want.

Celebrate instead the recovered, healed.

Bring to Light the Light bearers, and we all shall be healed together.

1.13.21

"The Perceptive Nature of Safety and True Trust"

True safety is not just assured but felt, wholeheartedly. It is a rested ease in equal parts unknown and innate spontaneous knowing. This is very different than the safety that is repeatedly assured by the carefully constructed medical institution.

When I go to myself, I check where I feel safe. The safety I feel around Hospital is instant and some kind of relief. But follow it through. There is a dark holding energy that shadows even the illusion of instance relief. It is not trust, but the opposite—and to giving up all faith in God in favor of the responsibility falling squarely on other shoulders, not mine (but I repeat, not God's). There can be instances where the heart is guided to seek what "they" offer by necessity, but most do not need that. Most are truly safer in the comfort of the home, where they can move without intrusion and Bloom without being plucked.

When I go to feel the safety of the home for birth, for me—I feel a steady opening and a deep, refreshing, fulfilling nourishing breath—like my body was waiting for my mind to ask and yes, yes it is not just safer but safe to birth at home, unassisted and undisturbed. It will probably go too fast and then I will miss it and want to turn back time. It is a gift, a miracle given, a true blessing. And yes, that, is true safety. The safety of the unknown and the innate knowing, that arising spontaneously directly from the Source to the birth in partnership, in loving communication between mother, child, and God. ♥

I honor the birthshaman within me. I act according to her wisdom.

I asked the baby what she is here for—her Purpose. The answer is:

Forgiveness.

It feels like a new truth, light—very powerful, opening in me. Pure, innocent, brave, strong, powerful forgiveness.

Light amongst the shadows.

Rainbow in the showers.

Bloom amongst closed flowers.

Blessed Light, completing the circuit through forgiveness.

What a blessing. I feel so much gratitude. And my crown chakra opens as the truth opens the birth canal for the birth shaman and for the baby (great grandmother's name, grandma's middle name, sister's middle name, mother's chosen name, forgiveness of all)

She is uniting our maternal family line through birth— the fractured females we have been—no longer alone, but together now. (No more competition but instead community togetherness through birth)

(I cry wholly and deeply, with Gratitude)

Listening to Yolande's freebirth affirmations and feeling deeply soothed, safe, trusting, grateful. Cool tears down my cheeks.

You never lost me.

I just found myself.

Deep breaths to shaman mantra. Drinking water. Reiki self-healing.

I forgive all those who have done anything that support my healthy natural birth process. ♥

I anticipate joyfully the beginning of my birth process as decided by baby and body.

I had a perfect pregnancy.

I had a perfect free birth.

I have a perfectly healthy baby.

I'm so grateful.

♥

It's the due date, and I'm having lots of adrenaline rushes. Trying to cope. Feels like a theme park—roller coasters one after the next.

It's late night on my due date, and I'm officially done being pregnant. I am completely ready to release this experience and transition to a life with my new daughter, outside of my room and in my arms.

I feel wholly unsupported by her father and perhaps that is because he can go no farther or further in this journey with us. It is now just she and I who can go deeper and travels the first canal together. I cannot blame him for being male.

He cannot fathom the depths of this holy feminine experience. These words try and yet it is in a place without words where the true sacredness of the sacred portal can be touched. I yield to the wisdom of the birth shaman within me now. And I do not even comprehend the vast reach of God's hand and this all. It's time to receive and be given.

I am worthy of the birth I have chosen ♥

Last night I saw a vision of the first shaman with blue light flowing through my crown and lit her face I heard a song "are you ready?" By princess and the frog. And as I fell asleep I saw psychedelic rainbow colors. When I woke up, I felt dizzy. I felt warmed by it as a sign of early labor. My partner felt that too and is being really supportive today. I

just ate some oysters and seaweed for the fifth time in 3 days, and only time in my pregnancy. I'm ready for this birth.

So grateful it is near and I will be able to freely birth and nurture and have baby in my arms.

"Soon I'll be holding my baby feeling only love and ecstasy" Yolande

Felt cramps last night. This morning feeling a little rings of passing energy sensation around vagina. Like ripples in a pond.

"Birth will pass through me like a cleansing rain."
Yolande

I am now safe to give birth to this baby.

I'm worthy of the birth I choose.

Everything is happening to support my free birth. Soon, I will have baby in my arms and feeling ecstasy and relief. I will call family and share the good news.

Big breath feels ecstatic.

Looking forward to giving birth can be like looking forward to a birthday. It will come and be magical. You will be celebrated. There's no need or place for anything but love and gratitude.

"My cervix is opening like a flower. Each sensation is a surge of power connection and love"

Love flowers with each wave washing over and threw me using the process and cooling the heat of transformation to a white-hot white light cooling flow.

"I am joyful, at ease and relaxed."

Ready to move between worlds to learn what I need in this lifetime to be the best mother and woman I can be.

Already feeling need for patience gratitude trust in God love Universe to be applied always every moment.

TRUST in God.

"A Note on Prodromal Labor"

Part of me loves the on and off nature of this prodromal labor I have more than enough time to satisfy my experience of this stage and every sensation prepares my body to have a more comfortable and smooth and quick labor—so it's work well done. That will better open me to the gentler spiritual side of the active labor transition and the actual birth moments.

Today I'm going to ecstatic dance, and that may be the very ritual to move this baby into this world powerfully and completely.

I painted yesterday. Got the idea to start a movement of "Labor Art"... Would love to see what women come up with. It's an inspired time.

After dance I got this feeling like what if I have been in labor and the baby is close to crowning?!

Anger coming up: the one thing I explicitly wanted was to not go past my due date. For baby to arrive before or on my due date. I couldn't do that. I control nothing in this birth, except my reactions to everything that happens. And for that I must go to surrender and love. Go into the pain until it becomes love. How can I be angry at God for bringing to me what I truly want, a healthy baby from my healthy body and divine timing? Trust. I can only be grateful ♥

Lots of strong contractions last night, just slept through. A little bloody show, just the famous speckles but enough to encourage.

But this morning back to intense emotional labor. Am I the only one who experiences birth like this?!!

MLK Jr Day 1.18.21

Those of us who have ever been made to leave at home we can relate to our children. Perhaps it is as if my child is being asked to leave the safety of my inner world and hers for an unknown outside. We know that if we fully trust in life are security and housing will be resolved and in fact we are set to receive everything we are willing to accept.

To our children dear angels of true source please surround us and our children and bring us comfort at this time and all time during every birth and every uncertainty that we ever experience in life. Sometimes we may be in the eye of the storm and being pulled out is that what it's like to be between worlds? Is it primal, ancient fear that's trying to move through me?

To know that we are safe and our children are safe? Are we all meant to go into the unknown with love and our hearts and to shed the fears for all the generations before and after us? Can I now realize that my mom was too afraid and my sister and my grandma, too, to trust the unknown of our very own bodies into the rebirth of birthing. And now I let go of all their projections and conjectures. And release them and us and me and we together.

This is not light. This is not perfect. This is the vomit of lifetimes of hiding from my raw primal power coming up for release. This is primordial fear. I am touching it. And it can transform me and I let it. I say yes.

Just recorded a podcast on addiction as that's what's authentically been a rising for me. Got honest and felt released. Had a contraction just after. Lots of nausea. Feeling depressed, lethargic, antisocial, hopeless—if that doesn't describe my adolescence I don't know what does. Is pregnancy a regression to help me to have a do-over for how I act in the face of these obstacles/opportunities?

need to be more active, but dance yesterday and slept so exhausted after. Still tired.

How to bloom? God will do it I need to trust. To believe. Every sensation even nausea is my body preparing for perfect birth.

Remembering

I don't need to know or learn anything in order to give birth. I listen to my body's cues. And I ride the waves of ecstasy as they move my baby from one world to our world.

This will happen in perfect timing.

1.18.21 4:30pm

My 2-year-old just howled out of nowhere. Like a baby wolf. Definitely getting close!!! (At this time I had no idea that I was still about a month away from the birth...as I write this now, she is 6 months old)

Emotional Labor Map

"How to navigate emotional labor"

Abandonment: Relate to baby. Baby must leave the comfort of the wound and trust. We must trust now too in a greater good beyond any being that feeds us life wherever we are. Mantra: I can trust this perfect process.

Loneliness: We can remember that right within our bodies is another soul beside our soul. This precious gift of life has chosen us specifically. And even when we cannot hear them, they are aware of us and loving us.

Mantra: I am being supported every moment, including now.

Sadness/Depression: Sinking feeling wave contraction may occur at any time and have thoughts attached to it of what is "causing" the sad. These thoughts seen from another perspective can also lead to calm, joy, ecstasy. Envision a white light at the peak if the wave. Allow it to expand beyond perception. Then allow yourself, within that Light, to find one way to be grateful (an aspect) for the occurrence of person or situation that has triggered the sadness. Then focus on that and relax the eyes and eyebrows and whole forehead and head and behind the ears and has and throat and breathe deeply into that gratitude, breathing out any

lingering shadow of sad. Response is gratitude. "Everything is happening by Divine Orchestration. The Universe is supporting me completely and wholly through even the smallest detail of my life."

Being Loved/Belonging: We are connected to many who we do not see, including an unconditionally loving true source, at all times. Also the support of our ancestors and angels surround us. And more so, we are connected to all women and mother Gaia and the birth process. We are receiving guidance and in ethereal hug at all times. We can always trust that, and relax into it, knowing the right guidance will come at any moment needed.

Primordial Fear: Deep breath. Release with exhale. Except the rhythm. Stop trying to control the feeling. Feel the surface below and around you.

Mantra: I am safe. I am connected.

Calmness/peace/euphoria: A soothing river of God's Love flows over and through us at all times, offering us everything we need and all of our heartfelt desires. We have access at all times. We only need to pause and allow our consciousness to drink of the waters to be revived.

Anxiety: Physical movement, changing locations, creating something, like a podcast, writing.

Mantra: baby will come in perfect timing

Excitement for Changing History into Her story: An adventure is unfolding within us. Life is being created. There is so much to be grateful for. There are so many opportunities as the blessed support of our new family member transcends from the spiritual to the physical manifestation of our child. And our voices are being expressed anew to reclaim this sacred passage is to life as ours, as we know it to be, deep within ourselves. This is an epic moment as the world is awakening to our gifts through the very experience that usher in trust and alignment with our inner purpose. It's an organic, natural unfolding. A bloom.

Lethargy: Rest. The body is preparing for work. Do not resist. Rest as much as desired. Remember nutrition and water.

Mantra: I am my beautiful body.

Relax: Deep breath. Yes. This moment of calm, peace, even joy is enough. Just to be here, perhaps relaxing in a warm epsom bath of lavender with chamomile tea, a candle and a book by our side. We are creating life! We deserve as much peace and quiet as we desire.

Hopelessness: Self-love, acceptance of humanity alongside divinity. Comfort from friends, loved ones, online groups, positive birth stories.

Mantra: birth is natural. This body and baby are wise. I can trust this process of birth.

Peaceful/Supported: Knowing we are born to birth and Any thought to the contrary is imagined or faulty reasoning passed down from generations of subconsciously adopted as thought patterns that are not true. We can rest and feel grateful for the work our bodies and our babies are doing, naturally, without intervention, just as a baby is formed in the womb without human instruction and instead through natural inherent, biological ability—freely given by God. And we can safely and comfortably rest in that true name everything comes in right timing, including babies.

Stagnation: Watching free birth videos. Reading positive free birth stories. Deep breaths. Movement— stairs, circle 8 on birth ball, walking.

Mantra: I trust the process of birth.

Inner heart knowing and connected guidance: in this blessed age we have full access to storytelling in any direction we choose. We may choose the direction of support and be vastly empowered by other mothers free birthing and giving life to our dreams before us. As we read or watch, our brains consume the reactions of actually experience. That can be of immense advantage to align us. Avoid the negative stories and influences. Tap into what you foresee for yourself. Allow your community to guide you through their steps (share resources). And as you do, be present with your experience and witnessing these achievements and interact from your heart and gratitude and observation of those who come before you, like spiritual elders. Next you will share your story and be the inspiration for someone else who like you needed that extra branch of support to enable her consciousness to fully accept and blueprint the miraculous nature of freebirth that lives us all. It's a community reclamation of true womanhood. And we do it best together especially in purifying and cleansing out any extra thought patterns that do not serve our hearts nor are higher purpose.

Pain: Deep breaths. Going into the sensation (not pushing it away), meditation.

Mantra: every sensation is bringing this baby closer to my arms. The stronger my sensations are, the happier my baby is.

Ecstasy/Euphoria/Pleasure: Our bodies naturally create \happy hormones. During the birth portal, those natural soothers are created in super-production. We can trigger their release into our bodies

Discontent: Sometimes when we do not like how things are happening, it's best to begin at accepting them. From there we are in the best state of mind to make good decisions based on our true intuition. Even when everything does not seem to be perfect, it is happening in perfect Divine Timing and there are gifts in every experience.

Gratitude: We can be grateful for the things we love, the things we like, and the things we don't like. Perhaps that nausea means our baby is growing perfectly and our hormones are working better than ever. If we knew that, we would thank the nausea and take it gladly over the alternative. See, everything has a purpose. Being grateful for things we do t even know the reason for is where true transformation begins. We can be grateful, every moment in advance for a healthy child and healthy body, and that will draw that reality toward us as the positive thinking improves our mental and thereby physical health.

Rage/Anger/Feeling of I can('t) do this/Blame/Fire: let it be encapsulated by Divine love, cooling and white, and become the fuel that propels me into greatness. To bring the baby in love. This comes up when triggered and attachment to someone for the causation occurs,

which can be only seeming, because ultimately we are
all responsible for our own emotions. The healthy
response is release and gratitude.

When we release anger and any attachment to anyone
(including self) or anything, it has nowhere to go but
down into the earth and expanding out to the infinite. It
can no longer stay with us and will be released and
therefore transmitted as an experience of ecstasy.
That's why they say forgiveness serves the forgiver most
of all, releasing us from a pattern of holding negativity
into expansive awareness and even receptivity. Rescue
remedy flower essence three sprays under tongue.
Mantra: I let go of what I think I know. I am open. I am
grateful for each contraction (emotional and physical)
as it brings me closer to baby. Mantra: my body is
capable of amazing things. I am loved.

Release and Gratitude: Being grateful for anything is
easy when we remember what really matters. We can
release attachment to what we think we know. We can
be grateful for contractions/waves because they
absolutely bring us our baby, and then they can become
a celebration each time. We can go beneath blame to
be grateful for the person underneath the blame in
whichever way they have and do serve/d us. We can
remember what really matters within the emotional or
physical waves, the spiritual spark at the center of it all
and be lit up and resolved in living harmony. From
there, solutions weave themselves all around us,
organically, naturally, guided by Divine Intelligence.

Courage: always trusting inner guidance no matter what it says. Corazon in Spanish is heart, and courage us about heart.

Pressure to Deliver: The mainstream dialogue about birth wants it to be over and done with. That is not this offering. This is not to say it needs to be prolonged but to trust that our bodies and our babies are innately wise and will deliver the baby when the timing is right. This is a relaxation of expectation that is necessary, forgetting of time, and checking in internally, which requires some alone and quiet time, to see that everything is going according to Divine Will. Much much more often than not, we limit our birth schedule to someone else's timetable when nature has another plan indeed. And that can lead to unnecessary interventions, which are entirely preventable by relaxing. The key is to maintain healthy practices, especially drinking plenty of water and lowering stress at the end. I also suggest not telling people your due date. Everybody will ask, because somehow in this society our grocers and our mom's best friend and our mail carrier all feel they have a right to know exactly when and where our babies will be passing through our vaginas, but that is not indeed their right. It's good to practice saying, "I'm keeping the due date private." You can give a range, but it's better to avoid the whole thing to avoid the interrogative gauntlet that comes about when we divulge the date that was only ever a guesstimate by a flawed medical system anyway. With that pressure relieved, we only have to worry about ourselves and release our own expectation of what the birth process looks like. It is spiritual, and in that very nature cannot be conceived or conjured by the mind. The mind must surrender for the full spiritual gifts to bloom. The birth will happen, no matter what anybody says. They don't need to be the first to know and nobody needs to be right about when or how it goes down. That's all really a male chauvinist body conquering type mentality and will completely whitewash over the emotional labor and spiritual growth aspects on the birth. When we release the pressure of controlling when, the baby comes in Divine timing. At almost 41 weeks, I feel a strong contraction at having written that. The birth process is also a rebirth process for the mother, a new experience of surrender where the body becomes an instrument for something much more powerful than that which we rarely ever touch upon in this lifetime. It's time to receive, not just to "do" or "make happen". Baby knows. Our body knows. And we will know too, when the time is right. Fear can be a loud and irritating voice. Do not buckle to it. Go within and adhere to Love. Love will guide you in whatever action steps are necessary. Trust the same force of life that naturally sparked your baby into conception and formed her perfectly. That force is with you always. Mantra: My baby and my body know how to give birth perfectly at the perfect time. I trust that baby will be born in the exact right moment.

"Time is irrelevant. Time does not exist. There is only this moment, right now."

To help labor progress: relax. Enjoy time with family. Up oxytocin levels by smiling lots.

The meditation referenced by Yolande is available at www.freebirthsociety.com That website also has many wonderful audio birth stories that I listened to throughout my pregnancy.

Another important resource that educated and connected me with Mamas honoring the sacred process was the Facebook page Freebirth/ Unassisted Childbirth as well as the book Birth on Your Own Terms by Heather Baker. She also is available as a traditional midwife and even assisted me with a call after the birth to let me know everything looked normal.

1.5.21 - 38 weeks 4 days

This time in my pregnancy feels like being in the eye of the storm. I am calm. I am peaceful. I am grounded. I am aware. It seems like many things are popping up to try to trigger me, but i am unphased. I am powerful. It feels surreal. I definitely feel like a portal. Some creative force is flowing through every cell of my being and out. One of these days is going to be my second daughter's birthday.

The mantra that came to me last night, in addition to being guided to breathe deeply during birth is: My body is capable of amazing things. And it feels good.

1.11.21

[An exploration of her name, which came to me clearly and has many meanings that continue to unfold. Part of her name mean ring, and she carries the same name as her great-Grandmother, which completes and cycles a powerful Divinely feminine connection and force back into the present moment, here and now.]

2.5

"For Baby"

Thank you for coming

on your time and mine

my mind has been running to find you this time

But our hearts were destined to walk one in one

hand in hand was the lesson patience for both from
both in Love

The way that you entered

the earth plain with me

kept my heart centered

kept my heart free

I will never be the same now that you're in my life

remembering just how

we soared through that strife

A journey together

began at the start

We chose each other

Our hearts chose our heart

1.20

The freebirth went BEAUTIFULLY. Huge great breath of relief!!!!!!!

(that was an affirmation...still 3 weeks away unbeknownst to me at the time!)

"I love my uterus so much. I feel in Love with my uterus right now."

thank you. you're doing great.

a day or two ago the birth shaman became clear and stern and serious. Today she looked happier and lighter. And just now she was moving all her hands around my crown chakra like moving the energy and clearing the space.

in this birth portal it feels like there us lots of healing energy. I am letting it go to lots of parts of me like my eyes and throat to help me be a better person. and any area I felt needs energetic support like lips.

breathing deeply certainly fuels the necessary contractions. water too.

Over previous days birth shaman...

looked up and stern

then looked smiling

then looking like moving and waving my crown chakra energy with feathers or hands then looked like flickering like electric

then looked celebratory like firework light

now nodding in reverence

1.20.21 later

she's holding the baby now

holding the baby in the shadows

now the baby is lit up from a heart spark and orbs of
light are radiating from her,

1.21.21 3pm

she says, "I will come soon. You can trust that Mommy. You are safe."

The baby has testable two orbs of bright light yellow white light auras around herself, the second outer one overlaps and connects with the spark of the birth shaman. I feel Love flowing into me from the connection. 5:09pm 12121 it's a portal I can go into like a cocoon and feel safe. we are a constellation, connected through Light. I can feel the part of me that doesn't want to let her go. in the birth shaman. holding her back. because I love our closeness so much. she is so special to me. I am crying.

I pray to release holding, dissolve contracts, release her to the earth. she does not belong to me but to true source. the earth is blessed to hold her now. I pray to let go

[6.24 Again, the underlines words seem to share a hidden message for us, all of us:

she says, "I will come soon. You can trust that Mommy. You are safe."

The baby has testable two orbs of bright light yellow white light auras around herself, the second outer one overlaps and connects with the spark of the birth shaman. I feel Love flowing into me from the connection. 5:09pm 12121 it's a portal I can go into like a cocoon and feel safe. we are a constellation, connected through Light. I can feel the part of me that doesn't want to let her go. in the birth shaman, holding her back. because I love our closeness so much, she is so special to me. I am crying.

I pray to release holding, dissolve contracts, release her to the earth. she does not belong to me but to true source. the earth is blessed to hold her now. I pray to let go

"You are white light, Love flowing, a portal, we, a constellation, of me, she. She, the, is blessed. Go!"]

The birth shaman is lit up, the chakras from heart throat ajna and crown now glowing like a constellation of stars from the baby. Also in half circle to left and right if each. feathers lit. alive.

I say her name over and over.

My belly contracts. She stretches and moves.

I see a fiery yellow spirit of a toddler running toward me over the bridge jumping onto me then holding my hand and we walk back toward the physical together. The birth shaman crown is lit and strands of light flow out of it through the top past the feathers up high like a fourth of July handheld sparkler.

I feel relieved. like I have let go of some part of me that was afraid. she'll come soon. and when she does it will be quick and easy. no one could have let this go but me.

it was me all along holding her back. it never had to do
with anybody else.

1.22.21

She is all lit up, the birth shaman, a radiant hazy glow about her feathers like a thick rounded arrow of light pointing up from the baby.

Tonight after the bridge walk the face of the birth shaman is lit up. A second woman. as if to draw my attention to her and direct me to her guidance. Perhaps I need to listen now. Silently. She began looking into my crown chakra facelit and wafting and waving it open quickly and dancing in circles. I felt my crown open. Still do. Feels trippy and tingly and open. And feeling some contractions. As above so below. She smiles. And nods. Crosses her arms. As if it say it is done. I breathe a sigh of relief. ∞

1.23

11:57pm birth shaman eyes are glowing bright today.
focused white lights.

1.24

Woke up full of energy. The birth shaman became a tree
of life with many light sparks as fruit, my ancestors all
supporting the freebirth. I feel calm, happy and grateful.
and full of life, energized. 6:07am, family numbers.

Freebirth Mantras

I have a beautiful, healthy freebirth baby and I am healthy and happy too

I am so grateful to have given freebirth.

I am being supported by my ancestors.

Anyone who doesn't know is like a young soul learning, like a baby who cries and needs to be comforted and reassured and just Loved and held.

My baby will pink up and cry and be so vital and alive when she arises.

She is picking the perfect time to come, with my body and so that I am completely ready and will have the best freebirth I can imagine. We are fully prepared now. I relax into knowing this freebirth is happening now and I am being Loved completely through every moment of it. Freebirth is easy.

Freebirth is fun.

Freebirth is like skydiving. It just happens guaranteed. And I am filled with intense emotions and ecstasy all around it. Emotions are a good sign that my body is preparing for birth.

Freebirth is peaceful.

Freebirth is natural.

Freebirth is organic.

Everyone in the Universe is supporting this birth now. Strong sensations like this mean birth is happening perfectly. The baby is arriving peacefully and triumphantly.

I can celebrate this beautiful freebirth.

Freebirth is sacred.

Freebirth is connected.

My grandmother's grandmother's grandmother is supporting me energetically, Loving me and baby and showing a Light ahead of us.

I am moving between worlds.

Freebirth is joyful.

Freebirth is celebratory.

These are moments I will always cherish, a sacred welcoming walk with babe, an initiation for both of us. I breathe deeply in Love.

Freebirth is safe.

Freebrith is normal.

I remember that I am here because birth is natural. The body knows how to birth perfectly.

The body is beautiful and Intelligent with Divine Love and Guidance. I open like a flower blooming with new life.

My new family member is here. We will share many joys and loves together. We remember each other.

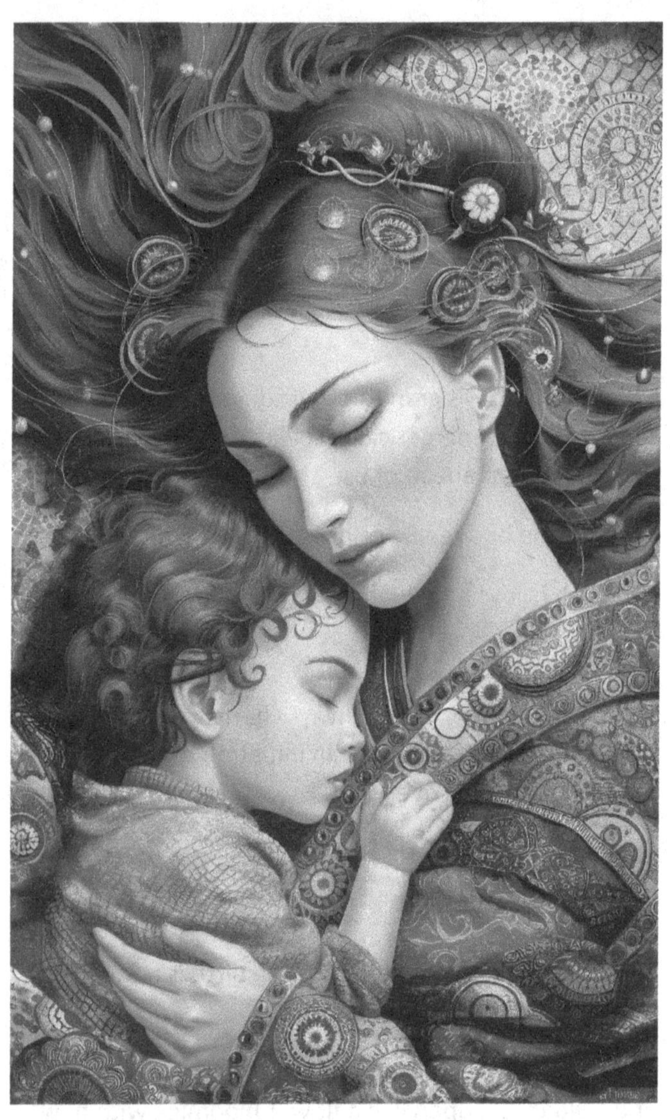

1.29

"Freebirth journal after it got easy"

I have a healthy happy freebirth baby.

Freebirth is easy.

My ancestors are supporting me wholeheartedly. The angels of True Source (God) are supporting me wholeheartedly.

Woke up full of energy.

6:07am, signs from my recently transitioned Dad and his Mom that they are supporting my choices. A book fell out of nowhere just now. Him again. A feeling a rush that he is so proud of me and in awe of my strength and courage, in my choice of sovereignty in this lifetime that he knows our family is growing together as i have committed to the evolution inherent in freebirth. Just a feeling.

Cleaning out the teacup and the tea leaves were a smile. A reminder and a congratulations in one.

I feel like I just turned a corner, and now it is flowing easily. I have done the emotional work necessary for freebirth, which for me was a lot, and now it comes as a gift from Grace.

Freebirth comes naturally and organically as a gift from Grace.

I am Loved Unconditionally and the birth blooms through me so easily.

Feeling ecstasy. Ecstatic tingles in legs. Seeing sparkles. Feeling surrendered to the Loving timeline whatever that is.

been relaxing more. and now after lavender bath feeling waves of ecstasy flow through me. music flowing. nature supporting. Called my brother who had always supportive. He is like a superhero in my life. My partner is being supportive now too allowing calm and quiet, nurturing, being kind and helpful.

birth shaman had looked like a tree cypress then eyes closed then war paint. now she looks like a bride, bedecked and glowing with light jewels and high feathers, lover and partner to God.

Who You Truly Are....The now is inseparable from who you are at the deepest level-Eckhart Tolle

Can't believe the full moon is today...it's after midnight...this is what my body has been preparing for my whole life. I am ready.

1.30

water gushed and I felt euphoria. amazing my body is
going in perfect timing, relaxed.

1.31

after an emotional evening, I self-healed while My partner channeled to me. During it I felt an enduring Unconditional Love with and from the baby. It was so beautiful, definitely from a long long time. So pure and strong. At the end, right after it completed, the baby in my tummy lit up with a beam of Light right through the center, top to bottom. I cried and shuddered and felt pure ecstasy and awe. It felt amazing. Like turning on a Light switch. Light something in the Universe had beenunlocked. Had a little bloody show this morning.

Going to ecstatic dance now. Feeling good and happy. happy hormones flowing.

yesterday

birth shaman innately decorated with white light stars today

birth shaman

1.31 11:22pm

has a half orb of white light stars stars geometry over
her crown up over me

2.1

lesson: do not impose will or expectation on this new being. listen and allow and trust they will feel what's best for all.

on the way to reflexology with dear friend Amy, I realized, "What if you knew this would be the best day of your life before it happened?" that's what this is. that's the power of freebirth.

Amy said I am the most powerful, vital and integrated person she has ever touched. pure communication between all body parts. she may have said strongest. she said the baby felt like stars, like pop pop pop and her hands motioned like fireworks.

2.4 I release

I release all fears related to birth.

I accept the control of the Divine and relinquish any control. I trust the baby and this body to follow the Divine Plan. Any thought that comes up and is not positive, I release, to be dissolved into the Earth. Any voices that I hear of anything not positive are not my own. They are not the Divine. I accept and release this reality so that my thoughts are Creative and Intelligent like the force that moves this body and this birth, I let go of all experiences in all lifetimes of birth and understand this is a new creative surge moving

through me, specifically for the perfect process of this baby and this body. I am reborn again in this lifetime with this new life who moves through me now.

Any fears or unsupportive thoughts that come up whatsoever are being released. I let them go as they are replaced with Love and Light.

Deep breath in the Love, full breath out the fear, and breathing in the Love again and again and again.

2.8

The irony of childbirth:

Miracle of Life,

Portal to the Divine

Gateway between body and Spirit,

New Spark beginning a new Destiny....

ummm....i just lost my mucus plug....began emptying my bowels...vomited breakfast....so....how long is this gonna take?

What a miracle that God formed a Life, from cell to completion, within your body for 9+ months! So who are you going to have do the birth for you, doctor or midwife?

You have another person INSIDE of you? And they are about fully formed and conscious? That's truly amazing...bet you can't wait til it's over, huh?

A heavy person walks by, nobody says a thing about their appearance. A woman with a big pregnant belly walks by, "Excuse me! Excuse me!!!! Yes, you. You're HUGE!! Due any day now huh?" Me: No. Stranger I've never met: "Oh then it's twins?" Me: "Nope." Them: "Oh but you're huge, big baby huh?" Me: "Nope. Regular sized baby. People's bodys are just different." Them: "Well that baby's cookin! (or some other quip)" Me: irritated, insulted, defeated, violated, rageful and most of all am thinking "my body is not your body."

2.9

Freebirth Playlist

https://www.youtube.com/watch?v=QVvW8iRtYnQSnat
am Kaur - Servant of Peace - Anandamayi Ma

https://www.youtube.com/watch?v=bIL881Nkbic Open
Your heart, Let the Love Shine

https://www.youtube.com/watch?v=SrF9PInr2wY Living
Sanctuary

https://www.youtube.com/watch?v=CqybalesbuA
Good Good Father

https://www.youtube.com/watch?v=Pm4kiRe-WWM
womb of the earth

https://www.youtube.com/watch?v=pBCUcx9iS5E May
I be Strong

https://www.youtube.com/watch?v=p4rRCjrAyCs Hills
and Valleys

https://www.youtube.com/watch?v=gbQ6Lfh5L14
Known
https://www.youtube.com/watch?v=w0gSMXEjgEk
Perfect

2.9 also...

Freebirth Books

Found this FREEBIRTH READING BOOKS list

- Juju Subdin's Birth Skills with Sarah Murdoch (Proven pain-management techniques for your labour and birth)
- Spiritual Midwifery (New stories and information 4th edition) by Ina May Gaskin

- Unassisted Childbirth (3rd edition) by Laura Kaplan Shanley

- Birth Matters (A midwife's manifesta) by Ina May Gaskin - Childbirth Without Fear (forward by Ina May Gaskin) by Grantly Dick-Read

- Placenta the Forgotten Chakra by Robin Lim - The Natural Pregnancy Book (Herbs, nutrition, and other holistic choices) by Aviva Jill Romm, MD

- The Essential Homebirth Guide (For families planning or considering birthing at home) by Jane E. Drichta, CPM & Jodilyn Owen, CPM

- HypnoBirthing The Morgan Method by Maria F. Morgan, M.Ed, M.Hy.

- Ina May's Guide to Childbirth by Ina May Gaskin - Emotions & Essential Oils (A reference guide for emotional healing (in pregnancy, birth and general health), 6th edition) no authors.

- Orgasmic Birth (Your guide to safe, satisfying and pleasurable birth experience) by Elizabeth Davis -

Birthing Your Placenta (The third stage of labour) by Dr. Sara Wickham & Dr. Nadine Edwards

- The Unassisted Baby (A do-it-yourself guide to pregnancy and childbirth) By Anita Evensen

Written 2.9

(3 days before birth)

43 44

All the voices saying you are not

good enough

do this

do that

I don't even want to say what they're saying

because I'm not alright

in my head right now

my body is flying sky high

feeling good

my baby is kicking inside

feeling good

my mind is a mess full of land mines

and the external devices of voices of people

preprogrammed to fear

in the world we live in right now and wrong here is
scrambling my thoughts so i don't know right from not
but

I

do,

I do.

I know deep inside with a voice that's not mine, but not
yours or the drones' or the trolls' or the crones',

I know I am well

feeling good feeling swell

how can i tell?

Because my body is thriving

my baby is alive and feeling like a bright light shining
and it's a silent communion

your head will never get

because it's well beyond the words

you try to fit on it.

And I'm angry and sad, you're cruel and you're mad. My
body is not your body.

This baby is not in you.

You do not get to tell this body or baby what to do and
neither do I

I tried, yes I tried,

buckled to your fear games,

poking and prodding

but it didn't work

and the rabbit hole you offer looks not the least bit
appealing

it in fact looks appalling.

So I love me right now

I love

I love baby right now

I'll be, just be, at 43

weeks right now

and not let y'all slaughter this one sacred cow, cause
every body is different

how can we be indifferent

to the cycles and rhythms

that sing our birth song in church hymns all life long?
My body

is

a church.

I am the sanctuary.

Please don't desecrate this alter of the war-washed and
wary. I

am

going

to

listen

this

time.

I am.

Trust is my new name.

And when I finish the fire walk, Blooming out from within, many more will follow

and they will do your fear in. Just you wait and see;

I trust this

Holy Fire

in me.

Birthday

2.12.2020

Lunar New Year

Day 1 for Her

Written 2.12

Tips for successful labor:

eat dates

drink water frequently'

electrolyte drink

poo often

get up and move when desired, alternating bouncing and opening hips and twirling on exercise ball

breathe deeply, breathe to anything not the best Yolande's affirmations

smile

oscillate hips while semi squat

move the way the body wants

relax jaw

(How it turned to true labor:)

When i got up, went to bathroom and thought about staying up or going back to sleep, the door to the room closed on its own so I took that as a cue to go do the labor work. (In bed before going to the bathroom) I had felt baby climb into place when I turned to the right and then again when I turned to the left and each time felt cramping contractiony thing so I felt like this could be it. the contractions become strong in waves and i flowed through them while watching portal movie and then affirmations by Yo. drinking water increased them. electrolyte drink. protein ball snack. bathroom clearing then mucus plug came out more. just got such a strong one i had to get up and move. moving helps/

drink iron Floridix drink

stairs

"the stronger my sensations the happier my baby is"

2.18 during "The Freeze" in Austin, TX

Texas freebirther here...gave birth at 44 weeks on the lunar new year 2 days before the water shut off, which has been for 5 days now, and i wanted to share some reflections with the freebirth fam and also open a dialogue for freebirth mamas in Texas. So please share your feelings if you are in Texas experiencing this as a new mama or soon-to-be (women who I know can and will get the freebirth they want and need). I think i often err on the side of toxic positivity, but in all honesty I would have to see this situation through clarity and I feel like a true warrior for a blessed cause. This current experience here has brought this realization more to Light, but I think that's the reality of where we FREEBIRTHERS are all now in this day in age. The system is stacked against us and we are a new breath of old wisdom in a confused age. I haven't had enough energy or presence to write my birth story yet, but it was not a pretty peachy birth that I had hoped for....it was raw and fast and messy. I needed those two days after birth to regain enough strength to be ok now. I had wanted the 40 days. I had wanted to honor this sacred portal I became. But I need to be clear with myself and with you, we are doing the real work right now. And this is what was asked of me.

Nobody has to have a hard birth; i think that's what many of us are here to say. But with my history and my family's history of birthing (systemized to say the least), this is what I was met with. And a freebirther who has an easy freebirth has done the work to get there and is just as much a warrior as someone who has any other variation of normal. I feel our community helps us to rise to this challenge. At some point in the many months I researched this stuff I saw that there are somewhere like a few thousand freebirths a year out of the 3-4 million births in the US...that is...that is almost hard to imagine. So that's the context. And every woman here is a warrior in the battle to shed Light on natural birth and reclaim our birthrite as mothers. One of the things I did prior to the birth was birth shaman meditations (the picture here is one i painted of the birth shaman last month). I kept checking in with her to see what state she was in—sometimes lit like a tree of life and sometimes slowly opening...but for the last week or so, she looked like a warrior, black streaks painted on her face and fierce with her long feather headdress. And then the freebirth happened in the way it needed to for my baby and me to ultimately be safe, and then the weather changed, almost like this baby and my body heralded this bright white Light that shifted everything around me...I truly believe all our babies do in this group.

So here I am, unshowered for 5 days, focusing on a newborn and 2 year old and working all day to get enough food and water and breastfeeding and naps for new babe, not sure if we would keep our power in the freezing weather, and my hair is the tangliest it has ever been like a literal birds nest—identical, unsuccessfully trying to keep peace with my partner and myself...and right after this huge argument because we are both stressed to the point of exhaustion, I paused and realized....I'm grateful. Grateful to be here following my truth and living this wildlife. To be happy and healthy and this baby to be as healthy as a month old or more holding her head up already and smiling all day long because she got a good birth and no vax nor vit k nor poking nor prodding nor stranger interaction nor any of that. I kept the freebirth secret from my Mom and brother and sister because I needed to be free of their programming, and when I told them yesterday, they were shocked to silence, and then they were proud and cheered me on. It was a big moment. This life is strange, but so magnificent. I love you all so much and am grateful for our freebirth tribe. You all have been so important to getting me here. And I want to cheer you on, where ever you are in the process. Please feel free to share any of your truth in the comments below.

Birth Story

(including birth history)

Birth is a natural process and can be fully expressed in divine order through guidance. It's only when there is intervention that the natural channel through which the birth is arriving becomes confused. These days, we need to trust our inner system regardless of what happens, always go in the direction that we feel is right.

It took me a while to coming around to writing this because so much has been happening and the intensity of the experience made me need to get some space from revisiting it. But here it is for posterity: a unique and heroic tale of the introduction of this human, named for her great grammy, into the world.

Those 44 weeks of pregnancy were the longest of my life. The last month stretched into a year, but ultimately I had to trust this body and this baby to bring her into the world safe and sound. And that's what happened, beyond all reason. Remembering that level of trust, I am reminded that this body is infused with God's essence of unconditional Love which can achieve anything, even the miracle of life and everything related. When we rest in Faith, miracles are possible. That's how birth is ever even started in the first place, with conception.

My first birth was an h birth, riddled with trauma and injustice. At 41 weeks I had been told my waters were low and if I refused induction I would be risking her life. I knew no better. I didn't know then that the fluid levels can replenish and actually fluctuate based on hydration. It was a scare tactic and I fell for it, full of fear, blind to my heart. I began pitocin the next day. Dozens of people put their hands in my body over the course of 40 hours of induced labor during which I was pumped full of pitocin and antibiotics. I got a balloon ball treatment and refused any pain reliever the whole time. Eventually, a terrible verbally abusive nurse came and my partner kicked her out. Right after she left I entered active labor. they had relentlessly checked me time and again and did not believe I could be that close, but all of a sudden I was at a 10 dilation and baby was on her way. Bloody show and water breaking on the toilet and ten people rushed in as I pushed with the waves I could see on the monitor. So many tubes and cords. Such a cold white room. So many strangers. Looked like robots everywhere. Two women felt kind, an African American woman and an Asian woman. Everybody else felt cold and hard and sterile. When the baby came out, the doctor insisted on manually removing the placenta right away. I didn't know I could wait and that it could come on its own in a few minutes if I sat up and went to a toilet and let gravity do the work. I didn't know I could take herbs to release it. They took my precious baby off my chest and the most painful part of the labor ensued as the doctor scraped and scraped, with scissors, for the most torturous 20 minutes of my life. After that I had to go to the surgery room to make sure there were no remnants. There were none. They took me from my daughter for the first precious hour of her life. I felt broken. I felt limp, defeated. But my next birth would help me to feel forgiveness and reclaim my body. I didn't know it could be so different.

We decided to give our daughter a sibling and became pregnant easily. I knew I wanted a different birth this time, so I opted for a midwife, whom I hired early without knowing how to research one. I never felt comfortable around her, and this only increased as each session went by—she gradually became less warm and more talking about worst-case scenarios. She told me one time, "you can't have all three—a good pregnancy, birth and breastfeeding—one has to be difficult!" UGH. WHY?! Another time she said, "do you want to sign the consent form for your husband?" and when I asked her why she said, "in case you don't survive the birth" or something like that...WHY THAT, TOO?! Bad vibes. Not what you want going in. She even explained all the terrible things that could happen to my placenta this time as if they

were status quo. And her list of supplies had tons of check gloves so even though the whole pregnancy she had not done one exam, apparently, she planned to ramp things up at the birth, without even mentioning or asking about it. Shady.

I only learned later that Traditional Midwives are the only real midwives. This lady I had paid $5000 to keep just because of the fear I had left over from my previous birth is known as a "medwive." They seem to be intent on reliving their past trauma in the experiences of their clients. Thank God the Grand Plan and my Faith stepped in and ousted her from any chance of being at the birth.

Here's how: I went long, very long. And as I crept into week 42, she ramped up her interventions and began incessantly bothering me when I needed to be the most focused and peaceful and safe feeling.

Holistic remedieserything except midwife's brew): Holistic remedies, miles circuit, walks, long hikes in nature, shinrin yoku, meditation, journaling, prayer, essential oils like clary safe, acupuncture, acupressure, eggplant, curry, spicy foods, slippery foods, healthy foods, indulgent foods, birthday party for baby, chiropractor (this one did work and came days before birth—first time I had been in this lifetime), flower essences, homeopathy...

It wasn't happening. In week 42, I agreed to have an ultrasound at home. They checked baby's movement, water levels, and one other thing I forget—I think the baby's overall health.

I had a wonderful reading. We both read healthy as could be. But the medwife kept trying to intervene and was pushing the midwife's brew, even saying you would drop it off and just hang the ingredients on my door after I ha said no, so I just stopped answering her texts for like two days and then...she dropped me. I was so relieved in my heart, like I should have let her go long before that. But I was a little aghast that she would suddenly check out like that. She said if I contacted her during the birth at all she would send an ambulance to me. She said she would still give us care for three weeks after as per Texas law, but I said no way! Our contract is over. I didn't want her near me or the baby. She was bad vibes through and through. I even did a ceremony to cut all cords and dissolve any contracts from any lifetime with her.

The whole time I had been checking in with me and baby and knew we were good. In the following two weeks I had ups and downs, many possible labors, and my waters even broke one time like ten days before and I was sure that was it....nope. Baby would come when she and I were good and ready.

I will add that during those extra two weeks I felt intuitively that baby was doing extra healing, that her body was repairing in ways that would not have occurred had I brought her out early.

She came out full of life and smiling. I'm so glad for the choices I made for her.

A day after starting to watch this movie called "Portal" on Gaia, and two days after my very first chiropractic appointment, I woke up at 4am and felt an urge to turn to

one side I never turned to because it was not the best side to lie in pregnancy. The very night before I had done a special prayer of surrender. I prayed, not to induce her, but to let go of anything I was doing to hold her in. I prayed with my whole heart. So that morning, when I turned, I felt her take both of her tiny hands and pull her head into my pelvis area and then I had a contraction. I then turned to the other side and had another contraction. I got up to go to the bathroom, and when I asked if I should go downstairs and try to make it happen or go back to sleep, the bedroom door slammed like someone was guiding me. I went downstairs, a couple of hours bouncing on my birthball and finishing the portals movie, and I woke up My partner. It was a pretty smooth couple hours there except when we tried to fill up the tub which did not work because we lived in an eco-community with low water allotment. Then transition came and I was screaming into pillows. And the next part was super fast, maybe 30 minutes. Going back and forth to the toilet (also known as the dilation station) to help the momentum keep up. I felt it had to happen fast. And it did. From 1 to 100 again. I couldn't believe—I felt inside and I was dilated and starting to feel the head, and then much more. Suddenly, I knew it was happening and I was like a wild animal needing to get somewhere dark and close together, like I cave. The only place in the house like that was the bathroom in the tub. I threw some towels down and got in there, standing up. So I stood there, crouched one knee down with the other leg straight, let my body push through the Fetal Ejection Reflex, and then switched sides. I was pushing, too, because I knew it had to be fast. I felt the ring of fire, the pushing happened, and out popped her head. My partner was so scared for me because of my breathing and sounds that he said he didn't even look. It's very visceral and men aren't used to that this day and age. And then, a pause, and the baby was pushed out. I caught her and rested her on the towels for a moment. I knew she would be fine and needed to just let my body have given birth for a second. She cried loudly instantly which was a wonderful feeling. I picked her up. I think her cord was wrapped around her shoulder or something and I untangled it—just naturally I was able to take care of that.

My partner thought she was a boy because of how her face looked which I think is hilarious, and

I saw she was a girl and was happy because that's how I had known her in the womb.

I was so happy to hold her. What a feeling to hold this precious being after all that.

And then, the part that the freebirth mother must attend to is the after. In sovereignty, she must look after herself.

So lots of blood clots came out, which I chalk up to my previous birth experience 100%. It's an understatement to say lots. And there was a bunch of baby poo, too, which is I think why I knew to give birth fast because there was none on her face just on the bottom part and coming out through the afterbirth, which means she was probably in the birth canal when the poop came out so she couldn't get any in her breathing passages.

I got up out of the tub with baby, and My partner helped me to lay down for a moment just outside on the blankets and towels. So I did, but then I knew we had to take care of the placenta. I was looking pale. My partner was trying to take video and i was like, "….no. I need to take care of myself now." I asked for the special scissors but he could only find the regulars so he sterilized them with alcohol and I cut her cord.

I set the baby on blankets and got up, but after a couple steps I immediately passed out really quick into his arms, which is why I recommend freebirthing with someone there to help if you feel called to freebirthe. I was alert immediately in sitting and checked my tummy to make sure baby was ok but then realized she had already been born, so I tried to get up again and the same thing happened again. My partner said, "What should we do? Should we call help?" I always knew that was an option, however, I knew what to do and thought there may be no difference in them helping me or not.

Anyway, I needed to follow my intuition. So I gathered my strength and told him to grab the tinctures and give me angelica immediately to release the placenta. I sat on the toilet, smelled peppermint to make myself pee, which worked and made room in there for the placenta to release. And it plopped right into the toilet. I grabbed a piece of it from the center that had not been touched by toilet water and put it under my tongue; I think I did this twice. I took the wombstringe for contraction inducing and pressed on my belly to help it contract. I also felt intuitively guided for My partner to grab the floradix iron drink I'd been on for weeks up until the birth and I took a couple big drinks, more than recommended but it felt right.

I later called traditional midwife and author of canonical freebirth book Heather Baker, in Guatamala at the time but she followed my updates and offered to help if needed, and I showed her pictures of my tum and fluids and she said I looked good and congratulations.

So this is the part where I say I'm not telling my freebirth story because it's perfect. To the contrary, I tell it because, I believe, given the level of physical trauma and scarring my uterus endured during the first birth as well as the duration of my pregnancy and the lack of physical fitness I had in my core area, that it's likely that if I can freebirth, most other women probably can as well. This does not mean any one person should freebirth.

I actually feel that regardless of the way a woman gives birth, as long as she is following her inner guidance and directing the flow of events in accordance with her heart's call, it is right. Always listen to the still small voice. Trust. If this account can do even one thing, may it embolden that voice into the fierce roar of the lioness within.

2024

She is almost three now. It is a New Year. I have decided
I am ready to share this story, in Faith, not because I will
ever be ready to stand in the Power of this Divine
Miracle that unfolded through me, but because
somebody out there needs me to tell it. Women are
being told untruths to frighten them into submission
when everyone should have a say in this all and
sometimes we know; we may sometimes know what is
truly best for us. And the conversation should be had at
the very least. The one with my side should not stay
silent just because Goliath roars a mighty roar. I don't
know how to show my face in this world as it is. I hope
and have Faith for something better. In the meantime, I
am Faith, and she is Her. And we are One with You
through it all.

As a coda for this storytelling, which I think my Dado
would like, I had a beautiful realization in rereading this:
the birth shaman, that was my Dado. I feel sparkles all
over as I write this, more than I have felt in some time,
and I cannot help but to smile. You see, after I gave
birth, I spoke with a psychic, and she told me that my
Dado may have never been able to hold my daughter he
would have known as more precious than life itself
while Dado was in his physical form, but he did hold her
while she was in my womb. I felt sparkles of epiphany
when the psychic told me this, as did another I told,
perhaps as do you. And now as I read this, somehow, I
recognize him in my own descriptions, even though I did

not recognize him when I wrote those words from years ago, and as I experienced this miraculous birthing process. My heart knew what it could tell me then, and here I am with a few years of wisdom and a panoramic view, and now, even when he was so close to me before, now with this distance, I see him there, helping me. And he still does. And he still holds us, and helps us all along the way. Just as all of our ancestors do, yours, too.

And this is where the story begins…

June, 2024, during an Eckhart Tolle retreat, I have finally gathered the courage to publish this. A person named Dawn messaged me yesterday:

"When the time is right, the Lord will make it happen."

Isaiah 60:22

The new way is not all we need, nor is the old. We need both. And we need both now.

The Light of Consciousness may enliven the new technology. There's nothing wrong with new technology; we have to make it right.

With every birth, we have
access to a portal of rebirth for
all of us.

ramcontent.com/pod-product-compliance
Source LLC
rg PA
7240726
008B/2590